GET YOUR DREAM TUMMY

A Comprehensive guide on

how to reduce belly fat

through healthy diets

SHAWN TAYLOR

Table of Contents

CHAPTER ONE

Introduction

A flat stomach isn't only good for your appearances; it can also help you avoid serious health problems like diabetes and heart disease. Unfortunately, due to the complexity of the human body, several factors (including hormones and heredity) can influence the degree to which your midriff is naturally flat. That's why it's a mental and physical challenge to try to reduce your stomach size.

Another problem is excessive fat storage. Even if you don't have a particularly large stomach, there are a number of things that might cause you to feel bloated and uncomfortable. The good news is that simple adjustments to your lifestyle can help minimize belly gas. Without resorting to harsh (and perhaps harmful) dieting methods, many of those modest behaviors can help you adopt safe, long-lasting lifestyle changes that will enhance your overall health and slim your tummy.

The diet plan in "Get Your Dream Tummy: Discover the Ultimate Diet Plan for a Flat and Toned Stomach" is meant to help you get your dream belly by giving you a holistic and long-term strategy for losing weight.

First, the diet highlights the role of nutrients in decreasing belly fat. It tells you what to eat to get a flat stomach and what to avoid if you want one. You can give your body what it needs nutritionally and energetically without stuffing yourself silly if you stick to the suggested meal plan and practice sensible portion control.

The diet plan emphasizes physical activity as a vital component in the quest for a flat stomach alongside proper nutrition. It offers a fitness plan that works in tandem with the diet, and it includes the most effective abdominal exercises. To get a flat stomach, you need to burn calories and build lean muscle mass through regular exercise.

The diet plan also places an emphasis on behavioral modifications that can aid in the reduction of abdominal fat. The body's innate capacity to burn fat and build muscle can be aided by taking steps to reduce stress, improve sleep quality, and maintain adequate fluid intake.

In sum, following this eating plan is a long-term solution to finally getting that flat stomach. It doesn't rely on fad diets or

other short-term fixes, but rather promotes a sustainable, well-rounded approach to health and wellness. If you stick to this strategy, you will not only get a flatter, toned stomach, but you will also feel better and live longer.

CHAPTER TWO

Understanding Your Stomach

Belly fat can be caused by a number of factors, such as a bad diet, inactivity, and stress. Losing abdominal fat is possible with better nutrition, more exercise, and other behavioral changes.

Abdominal fat is sometimes known as "belly fat." There are two distinct forms of abdominal fat:

- The visceral fat is the type of fat that surrounds the internal organs.
- Fat that is just below the skin is called "subcutaneous."

The fat right under the skin is called subcutaneous fat. It's the fatty tissue that gives when you pinch it. Subcutaneous fat may add to a pot belly, but it's safer than the more dangerous visceral fat.

Visceral fat poses greater health risks than subcutaneous fat does.

Many dietary and lifestyle adjustments can help people reduce their belly fat.

Excess fat around the middle is a health risk that cannot be ignored. Visceral fat is the sort of fat that builds up inside the abdominal cavity. It causes damage to the lining of your organs and can increase your chance of developing cardiovascular disease, diabetes, and several malignancies. When stored in the abdominal cavity, visceral fat can secrete inflammatory chemicals and hormones that play a role in the development of insulin resistance and, ultimately, chronic disease. Visceral fat is measured by medical imaging procedures like CT scans or MRIs because it cannot be felt or pinched.

Hormonal belly fat is a third type of abdominal fat that exists alongside subcutaneous fat and visceral fat. Women are more likely to experience hormonal belly fat due to hormonal abnormalities including insulin, cortisol, and estrogen.

The risk of developing a chronic illness can be estimated, and a targeted strategy for losing belly fat can be developed, if you have a firm grasp on the distinctions between the various forms of abdominal fat. Though both subcutaneous and visceral fat can contribute to a protruding stomach, losing the latter is more important for improving health and lowering illness risk.

Taking measurements of your stomach is an easy and accurate technique to monitor your loss of belly fat. A mirror and a measuring tape are all you need to determine your exact waist size.

How to take a belly measurement:

- Place your feet shoulder-width apart in front of a mirror.
- Wrap the tape measure snugly around your unclothed midsection, right above where your belly button would be. Make sure the tape is just tight enough.
- Make sure the tape isn't twisted or bunched and that it's lying flat on the ground.
- Inhale deeply, hold the breath, and then check the scale.

- To be sure of your numbers, take three separate readings and average them.

It is recommended that you take your waist measurement at the same time of day and with the same method each time to ensure accuracy. If you want an exact number, measure your stomach first thing in the morning, before you have anything to eat or drink.

Regularly measuring your stomach can help you see how your diet and activity are affecting your goals. An elevated risk of chronic diseases is connected with a waist circumference of more than 35 inches in women and 40 inches in men.

CHAPTER THREE

How to Lose Belly Fat with Food

Losing belly fat relies heavily on dietary changes. How much belly fat you have can be affected by what you eat, how much you consume, and when you eat.

If you want to lose belly fat with nutrition, the first step is to eat a healthy, balanced diet that's rich in whole foods. This means prioritizing fresh produce, lean proteins, whole grains, and healthy fats while reducing refined carbohydrates and added sugars.

Losing belly fat requires a combination of exercise and watching what you eat. Overconsumption of anything, even nutritious foods, can result in a calorie surplus and the accumulation of belly fat. Be mindful of your portion sizes and stop eating when you feel full rather than stuffed.

Tummy fat loss might be affected by when you eat. You should eat breakfast every day since it sets the tone for the rest of your day. Overeating and food cravings are both exacerbated by going too long without eating.

There is some evidence that a select few foods can aid in the process of losing belly fat. Fruits, vegetables, and whole grains, for instance, have been shown to help curb hunger pangs and keep you feeling fuller for longer. Lean meats, eggs, and lentils are all excellent sources of protein that will help you feel full and promote muscle growth.

Last but not least, if you want to lose belly fat, you need to drink plenty of water. Water helps flush out toxins and reduces bloating, both of which can contribute to a protruding abdomen, so it's important to drink lots of it.

Overall, losing belly fat requires a healthy, balanced diet with plenty of complete foods, portion control, regular meal timings, and water intake. Making these adjustments to your diet will help you lose belly fat and enhance your health and well-being in general.

What to eat and what not to eat to get a flat stomach

When combined with a regular exercise plan, the typical foods below can aid in your weight loss and belly fat loss efforts.

- **Resveratrol:** Fruits, peanut butter, and dark chocolate are rich sources of the antioxidant resveratrol. The accumulation of fat in the body is slowed as a result.

- **Darker red fruits:** are more successful in silencing fat genes. Some of the healthiest meals you can eat are red fruits like apples.

- **Choline:** Scientists think choline can silence genes that promote belly fat storage. Eggs are a good source of this vitamin.

- **Spices and Flavors:** Cinnamon and ginger, for example, may delay the activity of fat-storing genes and reduce inflammation.

- **Oatmeal:** Oatmeal is a healthy way to start the day, and if it's sweetened a little, it can also satisfy a craving for something sweet. Consuming high-fiber foods like beans, rice, oats, and berries can help turn off diabetes-causing genes by working with gut flora.

- **Extra plant protein:** Soybeans, split peas, and nuts and seeds including almonds, pecans, and sunflower seeds are all excellent sources of plant-based protein. You can up the calorie content of any smoothie by including a scoop of vegan protein powder.

- **Lean meat:** Keeping your metabolism revved up with lean meat is a good idea. Types of meat that are low in fat and calories include skinless chicken breast, turkey white meat, and lean cuts of beef.

- **Green tea, leafy greens, and colorful vegetables**: have been shown to lower inflammation and switch off fat-storage genes. Vegetables of various hues and textures liven up the menu. It has also been found that consuming green tea can help decrease visceral fat. Studies show that drinking green tea, which is low in calories and contains the fat-burning compound epigallocatechin gallate (EGCG), can significantly lower abdominal adiposity.

- Adding additional protein to your diet is another requirement of the low-carb lifestyle. Consuming a diet heavy in protein-rich foods like eggs, fish, seafood, legumes, nuts, meat, and dairy has been shown to reduce belly fat, boost feelings of fullness, and improve metabolic performance.

- Consuming more foods high in fiber will help you maintain a healthy weight. Vegetables and fruit, as well as legumes, oats, psyllium husk, and chia seeds, are all excellent fiber sources.

- Strains of the Lactobacillus family have been shown to aid in reducing belly fat, according to research. There was a 3% to 4% decrease in body fat after consuming yogurt made with this strain for six weeks.

- **Fish high in omega-3 fatty acids** are beneficial for lowering visceral fat. Two to three weekly servings of oily fish like salmon, herring, sardines, mackerel, and anchovies can considerably reduce liver and abdominal fat, according to a number of studies.

- Apple cider vinegar may help lower fat stores, according to some research. If you want to avoid having your dental enamel worn away by vinegar, diluting it with water is your best bet. Taking it first thing in the morning might help you cleanse your liver and drain out impurities.

To get a flat stomach, avoid these foods:

Foods that have been processed tend to have harmful levels of sodium, sugar, and fat. Inflammation and gas formation are possible outcomes.

- Carbonated soft drinks, energy drinks, and sports drinks are all examples of sugary beverages. They contain a lot of sugar and may cause weight gain in the abdominal area.

- Alcohol: Excessive alcohol consumption has been linked to both inflammation and abdominal obesity.

- Inflammation and gas are two symptoms that may result from eating fried foods because of their high levels of harmful fats.

- Foods that are high in sodium content include canned goods, fast meals, and processed meats. Water retention and bloating may result from them.

- Making these adjustments to your diet and putting an emphasis on healthy, whole foods will help you lose belly fat, feel better digest food, and reduce inflammation.

Planning meals and limiting serving sizes

The key to a healthy weight, including a flat stomach, is careful meal planning and quantity control. Tips for meal preparation and portion control are provided below.

Spend some time at the start of the week preparing for your meals and snacks. You can use this to plan ahead for a healthy meal and avoid making hasty, unhealthy judgments when hunger strikes.

Reduce Your Portion Size By Using Smaller Dishes Using smaller plates and bowls can help you feel as though you're eating more food than you actually are.

Use a Food Scale or Measuring Cups Make sure you're getting the right amount of food by using a food scale or measuring cups, especially when it comes to high-calorie foods like nuts, cheese, and oils.

To prevent binge eating and make it easy to grab a nutritious snack on the fly, pre-portion items into separate bags or containers.

veggies, especially a wide variety of colorful veggies, can help you feel full and satisfied while also supplying vital nutrients, so make sure they take up at least half of your plate at every meal.

Do not go too long without eating; this can lead to binge eating later on. You should eat three main meals and one or two snacks daily.

Enjoy your food by eating deliberately and appreciating each bite to avoid feeling hungry between meals.

Pay heed to your body's signals for hunger and fullness. Avoid mindless nibbling and stop eating when you're full.

The "half-plate rule" suggests filling half your plate with veggies, a quarter with protein, and a quarter with whole grains to help with portion control.

You may improve your eating habits and get a flat stomach by following these suggestions for meal planning and amount control.

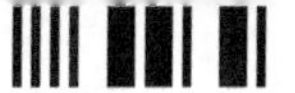

CHAPTER FOUR

The Best Diet for a Flat Stomach

How to Reduce Belly Fat in 7 Days with Food

If you want to reduce weight and get rid of belly fat, this 7-day eating plan is for you. Don't forget that this is only a sample menu and can be modified to fit your tastes and dietary requirements.

Day 1

Breakfast(290 cals, 4 g fiber)

- One Serving Muffin-Tin Omelets with Feta and Peppers,
- 1 average orange
- 8 oz. green tea

A.M. Snack(11 g dietary fiber, 214 kcal)

- 1.25 cup of fat-free kefir
- Raspberries, either fresh or frozen, 1 cup
- 2 tsp. chia seeds

Lunch (345 cals, 8 g fiber).

- One Whole-Grain Veggie Wrap per serving

Evening Snack (221 cals, 4 g fiber)

- One-fourth cup of spicy lime peanuts

Dinner(with 410 calories and 13 g fiber)

Baked Vegetable Soup, 2 cups

- 1/4 cup hummus spread on a toasted whole-wheat pita round, measuring 4 inches in diameter

Day 2

Breakfast (290 cals, 4 g fiber)

- Muffin-Tin Omelets with Feta and Peppers, per Serving
- 1 average orange
- 8 oz. green tea

A.M. Snack (11 g dietary fiber, 214 kcal)

- 1.25 ounces of fat-free kefir
- Raspberries, either fresh or frozen, 1 cup
- 2 tsp. chia seeds

Lunch (324 cals, 4 g fiber)

- Included: Spinach and Artichoke Salad with Parmesan Vinaigrette (one serving).

Evening snack (A 46-calorie, 2-gram-fiber.)

- Served on top of 1 1/2 cups of air-popped popcorn with 1 tsp. Spices from Italy

Dinner(630 kcal, 12 g fiber)

- Chickpea Pasta with Lemony Parsley Pesto, 1 3/4 Cups

Day 3

Breakfast (290 cals, 4 g fiber)

- Muffin-Tin Omelets with Feta and Peppers, One Serving
- 1 average orange
- 8 oz. green tea

A.M.   Snack210-calorie   (4-g-fiber) munchies

- 1 standard-sized banana

- 1 Tbsp. peanut butter

Lunch (324 cals, 4 g fiber)

- Included: Spinach and Artichoke Salad with Parmesan Vinaigrette (one serving).

Evening Snack (A 159-calorie, 11-g-fiber)

- One-half cup of fat-free kefir

- Raspberries, either fresh or frozen, 1 cup

- 2 tsp. chia seed

Dinner (446 kcal, 10 g dietary fiber)

- Chhole (Chickpea Curry), one serving

- One pita bread, whole wheat, six inches in diameter

Day 4

Breakfast (380 cals, 10 g fiber)

- Matcha green-tea latte, one serving size

- 1 slice of Avocado Toast with Everything on it

- A pair of kiwi fruit

A.M. Snack (just 1 g fiber and 113 calories)

- Muffin-Tin Omelets with Feta and Peppers, one-half serving.

Lunch (324 cals, 4 g fiber)

- Included: Spinach and Artichoke Salad with Parmesan Vinaigrette (one serving).

Evening Snack (221 cals, 4 g fiber)

- One-fourth cup of spicy lime peanuts

- Supper (453 kcal, 14 g dietary fiber)

- Roasted Root Vegetables and Greens Served Over Spiced Lentils, One Serving

Day 5

Breakfast (490 Calories, 18 Fiber)

One cup Kefir

- Three-quarters of a cup of plain muesli
- Three-quarters cup of fresh raspberries

Muesli and fruit go great on top of kefir.

- 8 oz. green tea

A.M. Snack (just 1 g fiber and 113 calories)

- Muffin-Tin Omelets with Feta and Peppers, one-half serving.

Lunch (324 cals, 4 g fiber)

- Included: Spinach and Artichoke Salad with Parmesan Vinaigrette (one serving).

Evening Snack (95 calories, 4 g fiber)

- One large apple

Dinner (497 cals, 8 g fiber)

- 1 serving of Spaghetti Squash and Chicken Pesto with Avocado

Day 6

Breakfast (296 kcal, 6 g fiber)

- Matcha green-tea latte, one serving size
- slice of Avocado Toast with Everything on it

A.M. Snack (just 113 calories and 1 g fiber)

- Muffin-Tin Omelets with Feta and Peppers, one-half serving.

Lunch (360 kcal, 13 g fiber)

- White bean and vegetable salad, one serving

Evening Snack (A 210-calorie, 4-gram-fiber)

- 1 standard-sized banana
- 1 Tbsp. butter on toast

Dinner (532 cals, 5 g fiber)

- Shrimp Paulista, one dish
- Brown rice, 1 cup, cooked; 1 tsp. minced chives
- Broccoli florets, cooked for 1 cup, with 2 tsp. olive oil, and sprinkled with salt and pepper to taste

Day 7

Breakfast (290 cals, 4 g fiber)

- Muffin-Tin Omelets with Feta and Peppers, One Serving
- 1 average orange
- 8 oz. green tea

A.M. Snack (200 calories, 5 g fiber)

- One large apple
- 1 Tbsp. butter on toast

Lunch (The 230-calorie, 11-g-fiber)

- White bean and avocado toast, one serve

Evening Snack (11 g Fiber, 186 Calories)

- Half a cup of fat-free kefir
- Raspberries, either fresh or frozen, 1 cup

- 2 tsp. chia seed

Dinner (with 605 calories and 8 g fiber)

- One dish of Chicken Hasselback Caprese

- One cup of brown rice, cooked

- 1/2 tsp. oregano, dried

Be sure to drink lots of water and low-calorie beverages like unsweetened tea and sparkling water every day. Sticking to this diet and picking healthy options will help you lose belly fat and feel better in general.

Methods for adapting the diet to individual tastes and needs

There are a few primary considerations when adapting a diet plan to fit a variety of lifestyles and personal preferences. Some suggestions for dietary tweaks are as follows:

Meal Plan Adjustments Vegans, those avoiding gluten, and those who are lactose intolerant may need to make adjustments to the meal plan. It may be necessary, for instance, to replace animal-based proteins with plant-based alternatives or gluten-containing cereals with gluten-free alternatives.

Calorie Requirements Depending on characteristics such as physical activity, age, gender, and other factors, calorie requirements can range widely. If you discover that the calories provided by the meal plan are insufficient, you can always supplement with snacks or eat more food.

If you have dietary allergies or specific culinary preferences, you may wish to make adjustments to the meal plan. You might, for instance, replace some of the recipes with ones for stir-fries or sushi bowls if Asian fare is more to your liking.

Time constraints: If your timetable is tight, you may need to make some adjustments to the meal plan. Doing so may entail things like discovering dishes that can be cooked in under 30 minutes or prepping food in advance.

If money is tight, you may need to make adjustments to the meal plan in order to make it more manageable. Possible substitutions include canned tuna or chicken thighs for more pricy options like salmon.

Keep in mind that the best way to improve your diet is to make changes that are practical for you. You'll have a better chance of sticking to the plan and accomplishing your objectives if you tailor your alterations to your specific needs and preferences. Consult a qualified dietitian or nutritionist for assistance in developing a healthy eating plan if you feel overwhelmed.

CHAPTER FIVE

Abdominal exercises

While a healthy diet is essential, working out can also help you burn fat and tone your abdominal muscles, leading to a flatter stomach.

Here are some great ab workouts that really work:

Plank: The plank is an excellent exercise for developing abdominal muscular tone and stabilization. To perform a forearm push-up, first assume a push-up stance and lower yourself to your forearms. Maintain a perfect line from your head to your heels for 30-60 seconds as you hold this stance.

Bicycle crunches: Bicycle crunches are an excellent way to strengthen your oblique muscles and define your waistline. Position yourself on your back with your legs bent and your hands behind your head. Raise your shoulders off the floor as you extend your right leg and bring your right elbow to your left knee. Turn around and do it again.

Russian twist: Another exercise that focuses on the oblique muscles is the Russian twist. Put your feet flat on the ground and your knees bent. Raise your feet off the ground and lean back a little. To strengthen your core, hold a medicine ball or weight in front of your chest and rotate your body to the left, and then the right.

Reverse crunches: Tummy flattening reverse crunches focus on strengthening the lower abs. Get on your back with your knees bent and your legs propped up. Raise your thighs off the floor and lower them back down carefully.

Cardio: Incorporating cardio into your program alongside specific ab exercises can help you burn fat and expose toned muscles. To raise your heart rate and burn calories, try activities like running, cycling, or swimming.

Keep in mind that the best outcomes can be attained by combining exercise with a balanced diet. In addition to a healthy diet and regular exercise, doing these abdominal exercises at least twice a week will help you get the flat stomach of your dreams.

Making an exercise schedule that works in tandem with the diet

To complement your diet and help you achieve your goal of a flatter stomach, you need put some thought into your exercise routine. If you want to create a training routine that complements your nutrition, consider the following:

Consistency: Maintaining a consistent routine is essential for getting a flat stomach. You should try to work in 30-60 minutes of cardio and strength training at least three to four times a week.

Cardio: The extra fat and calories you carry around your midsection can be burned off with cardio sports like running, cycling, or swimming. You should aim to do cardio at a moderate level for 30-60 minutes, three to four times a week.

Strength Training: Abdominal muscles can be toned and a flatter stomach can be achieved by strength training activities including planks, crunches, and Russian twists. Try to work in some form of strength training at least twice a week.

Recovery: If you're engaging in high-intensity exercises like weight lifting or high-intensity interval training (HIIT), you need to give your body time to recuperate in between sessions. Plan some downtime into your schedule so your muscles can heal and grow stronger.

Progression: Increase the difficulty or length of your workouts as your fitness level rises to keep your body challenged and your results coming. You can do this by incorporating more difficult cardio activities like sprints or hill climbs, or by raising the weight or number of repetitions in your strength training routine.

It's crucial to complement your exercise routine with a healthy eating plan for the best outcomes. A flat, toned stomach is one of the many fitness goals that can be attained by a combination of a healthy diet and frequent exercise.

CHAPTER SIX

Altering Your Habits to Lose Belly Fat

Reducing stress and getting better sleep are two of the most important things you can do for your health and to get a flat stomach. Some suggestions for relieving tension and getting a better night's rest:

- Reducing stress and increasing relaxation can be accomplished by regular practice of relaxation techniques such as deep breathing, meditation, or yoga.

- Maintaining a regular exercise routine might help with stress management and sleep quality. Do some sort of physical activity for at least 30 minutes at a low intensity on most days of the week.

- Create a Bedtime Routine Creating a bedtime ritual helps improve sleep quality. Maintain a regular sleep/wake schedule, even on the weekends.

- Stay away from screens at least an hour before bedtime, as the blue light emitted by smartphones, tablets, and computers has been shown to disrupt sleep. Put away the electronic devices at least 30 minutes before you turn in.

- Make your bedroom comfortable for sleeping by ensuring it is dark, quiet, and cool. To avoid interruptions, set up a blackout curtain, insert some earplugs, or turn on a white noise machine.

- Consuming caffeine or alcohol close to bedtime can make it difficult to fall asleep. Avoid using these substances as much as possible, especially at night.

- Don't suffer in silence if you need help coping with overwhelming emotions; talk to trusted loved ones or a mental health professional. Better sleep and wellness are two benefits that might result from reducing stress.

Stress may be reduced, sleep can be improved, and a healthy lifestyle can be supported so that you can achieve your goal of a flatter stomach by following these suggestions.

How drinking water can help you lose belly fat

In addition to being crucial for general health, drinking plenty of water will also help you shed unwanted belly fat. Some reasons include:

- Drinking enough water throughout the day might help you feel full and satisfied, preventing you from eating more than you need and facilitating weight reduction.

- In order to enhance the number of calories burned daily, it is recommended to drink at least eight glasses of water daily.

- Because the body retains water when you're dehydrated, drinking water can help alleviate the bloating and puffiness that result. Getting plenty of water in your system will help you eliminate excess fluid and feel less bloated.

- Hydration can aid digestion, which in turn can alleviate digestive issues including bloating and constipation.

- Hydration plays an important part in losing belly fat and in maintaining overall health. The average person needs between 8 and 10 glasses of water each day; more in hot weather or during exercise. Vegetables and fruits contain water, and so do herbal teas. Maintaining an adequate water intake will help you lose belly fat, since it aids in metabolism and digestion.

Alterations to your daily routine that will help you get the flat stomach of your dreams

Getting the flat stomach of your dreams requires more than just a balanced diet and regular exercise routine. Some adjustments to your routine can help you succeed:

- Reduce your alcohol intake; doing so may help reduce the accumulation of fat around your midsection. If possible, cut back on, or abstain from, drinking.

- Stop smoking; it's been linked to belly fat and many other health problems. Quitting smoking can help you have a flat stomach and enhance your health in general.

- Reduce your stress levels; being stressed might make you gain weight and cause belly fat. Include yoga, meditation, or deep breathing exercises in your regular routine to help manage stress.

- A good night's sleep is not only helpful for your weight loss attempts, but for your health in general. Get between seven and eight hours of sleep nightly to maintain a healthy metabolism and lower stress.

- Avoid overeating by paying attention to serving sizes and stopping before you feel full. To avoid feeling hungry again too soon after eating, try using smaller plates, measuring out your food, and eating more slowly.

- In addition to regular exercise, it's important to maintain a high level of activity throughout the day. Stand up and stretch every so often, take a walk around the block at lunch, or use the stairwell instead of the elevator.

You can help your attempts to lose belly fat and enhance your health by making these adjustments to your daily routine.

CONCLUSION

A brief summary of the information presented in "Get Your Dream Tummy: Discover the Ultimate Diet Plan for a Flat and Toned Stomach" follows.

Knowing the different forms of belly fat might help you choose the best method for shedding that stubborn fat.

Taking measurements of your stomach might show you if you're shedding belly fat and help you stay motivated.

Losing belly fat is largely dependent on dietary changes. Losing weight and belly fat can be aided by eating a good, balanced diet high in protein, fiber, and healthy fats.

A diet high in full, nutrient-dense foods and low in processed foods, sweets, and saturated fat may facilitate the removal of abdominal fat.

Guidelines for meal preparation and portion control: Keeping to a balanced diet can be aided by planning meals in advance and paying attention to serving sizes.

You can get a sense of what a diet that helps you lose belly fat would look like by looking at an example meal plan.

The diet plan can be adapted to accommodate various dietary needs and lifestyles, including those of vegetarians and those who avoid gluten.

Exercise can help you lose belly fat and maintain a flat stomach by increasing your metabolism and strengthening your abdominal muscles.

Making a plan for exercise that fits in with your diet is a great way to speed up your progress toward your goal of losing belly fat.

Managing stress and getting adequate sleep are not only important for your health as a whole, but they can also help you lose belly fat.

Water's function in helping you lose belly fat: It suppresses hunger, speeds up your metabolism, eases bloating, and promotes healthy digestion, all of which contribute to your overall weight reduction and belly fat loss efforts.

Reducing alcohol intake, giving up smoking, and increasing activity levels are just a few examples of the kinds of lifestyle adjustments that might help you get the flat stomach of your dreams.

Keeping yourself inspired and committed to your belly diet plan is crucial to your success. Finally, here are some pointers to keep you going:

You'll have more success staying motivated and making progress toward your ultimate goal of losing belly fat if your goals are reasonable.

Keep a food diary to keep track of what you eat and how it affects your progress in losing belly fat.

Find a support system: A friend or family member can be an excellent source of motivation and accountability.

Celebrate your progress along the way by treating yourself to something you want, like a new exercise attire or a day at the spa.

To keep yourself motivated and on track, it is important to keep a positive outlook and to pay attention to your successes rather than your failures.

Losing belly fat is a slow process, so give yourself time and don't give up.

Alternate your diet and exercise routine to keep things interesting and keep yourself motivated.

If you follow these last few guidelines, you should be able to maintain your motivation and stick to your tummy diet plan, resulting in long-term success and a flatter, more toned stomach.

THE END